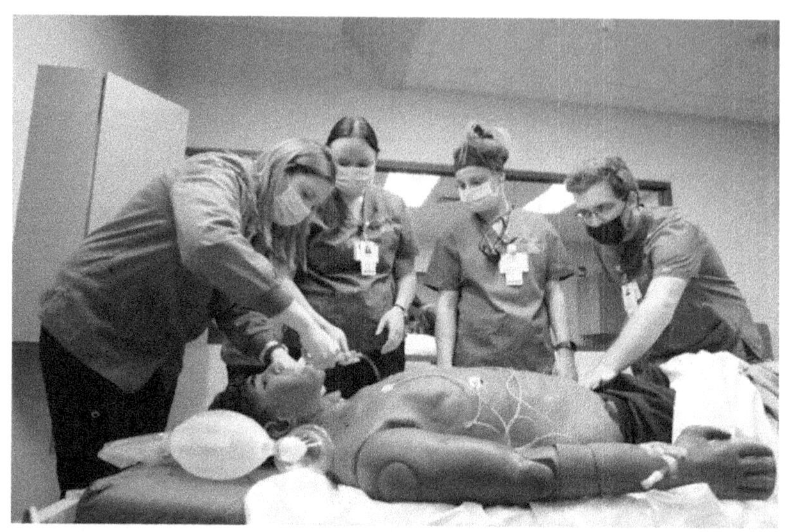

How to apply and get admitted to nursing school

RED DOT PUBLICATIONS

Chapter 1: Introduction

- What is nursing?
- Why become a nurse?
- The different types of nursing programs
- The nursing school admissions process
- Application fees

Chapter 2: Requirements for Nursing School

- GPA requirements
- Pre-requisites
- The Nursing School Admission Test (NCLEX)
- Other requirements

Chapter 3: Preparing Your Application

- Choosing the right schools
- Completing the application
- Writing your personal statement
- Getting letters of recommendation

Chapter 4: Interviewing for Nursing School

- What to expect
- How to prepare
- What to wear
- What to say

Chapter 5: Getting Accepted to Nursing School

- The waiting game
- What to do if you're not accepted
- Next steps

Introduction

Nursing is a rewarding and challenging career that allows you to make a difference in the lives of others. If you are considering a career in nursing, there are a few things you need to know about the application process.

In this article, we will discuss the different requirements for nursing school, how to prepare your application, and what to expect during the interview process. We will also provide some tips on how to increase your chances of getting accepted to nursing school.

Whether you are a high school student or a college student, this article will give you the information you need to start your journey to becoming a nurse.

Did you know that there is a shortage of nurses in the United States? According to the American Nurses Association, there will be a shortage of 1.2 million nurses by 2030. This means that there is a great demand for nurses, and if you are interested in a career in nursing, now is a great time to start your journey.

Context:

The nursing school admissions process can be competitive, but it is possible to increase your chances of getting accepted by following these tips:

- **Start early**. The process of getting into nursing school can take several years, so it is important to start early. This will give you time to complete the necessary coursework, take the NCLEX, and gain relevant experience.

- **Get good grades.** Your GPA is one of the most important factors in nursing school admissions. Aim for a GPA of 3.7 or higher.

- **Take the NCLEX.** The NCLEX is a standardized test that is required for admission to nursing school. It is important to score well on the NCLEX, as your score will be compared to other applicants.

- **Gain relevant experience.** Nursing schools want to see that you are committed to a career in nursing. Gain relevant experience by shadowing nurses, volunteering in a medical setting, or conducting research.

- **Write a strong personal statement.** Your personal statement is your chance to tell the admissions committee why you want to be a nurse. Make sure your statement is well-written and that it highlights your strengths and experiences.

- **Get strong letters of recommendation**. Letters of recommendation are an important part of your nursing school application. Ask professors, mentors, or other professionals who know you well to write letters on your behalf.

- **Apply to a variety of schools**. Nursing school admissions is a competitive process, so it is important to apply to a variety of schools. This will increase your chances of getting accepted.

By following these tips, you can increase your chances of getting accepted to nursing school and start your journey to a rewarding and challenging career.

Chapter 1: Introduction

What is nursing?

- Nursing is a vital profession within the healthcare sector that focuses on promoting, maintaining, and restoring the health and well-being of individuals, families, and communities. Nurses play a crucial role in providing patient care, advocating for patients' rights, and working collaboratively with other healthcare professionals to ensure optimal outcomes for those in need.

- The primary responsibilities of nurses include:

- **1. Patient Care:** Nurses are directly involved in providing care to patients, including administering medications, monitoring vital signs, dressing wounds, and assisting with various medical procedures. They play a pivotal role in ensuring patients' comfort and safety during their hospital stay or medical treatment.

- **2. Education and Support:** Nurses educate patients and their families about their health conditions, treatment plans, and self-care techniques. They provide emotional support and help patients cope with their illnesses or injuries, fostering a positive healing environment.

- **3. Health Promotion and Prevention:** Nurses work to promote healthy lifestyles and disease prevention. They provide information on proper nutrition, exercise, and immunizations, as well as identifying potential health risks within communities.

- **4. Collaboration with Healthcare Team:** Nurses collaborate with physicians, therapists, and other healthcare professionals to coordinate patient care. They contribute valuable insights, observations, and assessments to ensure the best possible outcomes for patients.

- **5. Advocacy:** Nurses serve as advocates for their patients, ensuring their needs and preferences are communicated and respected throughout the healthcare process. They act as a bridge between patients and the healthcare system, making sure patients receive the best care possible.

Nursing is a diverse and dynamic profession, offering various career paths, including specialties in areas such as pediatric nursing, critical care, gerontology, psychiatric nursing, and many more. Nurses can work in hospitals, clinics, long-term care facilities, community health centers, schools, and even in patients' homes as home health nurses.

The nursing profession requires a high level of compassion, empathy, critical thinking, and problem-solving skills. Nurses undergo rigorous education and training, often earning degrees such as Bachelor of Science in Nursing (BSN) or Associate Degree in Nursing (ADN) and obtaining licensure through exams specific to their country or state. Throughout their careers, nurses make significant contributions to the well-being of individuals and communities, making them an indispensable part of the healthcare ecosystem.

Why become a nurse?

Becoming a nurse is a deeply rewarding and meaningful career choice that appeals to individuals for a variety of reasons. Here are some compelling reasons why many people choose to become nurses:

1. **Passion for Helping Others:** Nursing attracts individuals who have a genuine desire to make a positive impact on people's lives. Nurses have the opportunity to provide care, support, and comfort to patients during times of vulnerability, illness, or injury, making a significant difference in their well-being.

2. **Job Stability and Demand:** The healthcare industry continues to experience strong demand for nurses worldwide. As the population ages and healthcare needs increase, nurses are in high demand, leading to job stability and various career opportunities.

3. **Diverse Career Paths:** Nursing offers a broad range of career paths and specializations. Whether one prefers to work in a hospital, clinic, school, research setting, or even as a travel nurse, there are diverse opportunities for growth and professional development.

4. **Personal Fulfillment:** Nursing provides a sense of fulfillment, knowing that one's work directly contributes to the improvement of patients' health and quality of life. The gratitude and appreciation from patients and their families often reinforce the value of a nurse's role.

5. **Continuous Learning:** Healthcare is an ever-evolving field, and nursing offers the chance to engage in lifelong learning. Nurses are encouraged to stay updated with the latest medical advancements, technologies, and evidence-based practices, keeping their skills sharp and knowledge current.

6. **Team Collaboration:** Nurses work closely with other healthcare professionals, creating a collaborative and supportive work environment. Teamwork is essential in healthcare, and nurses often find camaraderie and support from their colleagues.

7. **Flexibility and Mobility:** Nursing credentials and licenses are often transferable between states and countries, providing nurses with the opportunity to work in different regions or even explore international nursing opportunities.

8. **Challenging and Dynamic Work:** Nursing is a profession that requires quick thinking, problem-solving, and adaptability. Each day brings new challenges, ensuring that the work remains engaging and dynamic.

9. **Job Satisfaction:** Studies have shown that nurses report high levels of job satisfaction. The ability to positively impact the lives of others, along with the sense of camaraderie among healthcare professionals, contributes to overall job satisfaction.

10. **Competitive Compensation:** Nursing offers competitive salary and benefits packages, which can vary based on the level of education, experience, and specialization.

Overall, nursing is a calling for those who are dedicated to caring for others, making a real difference in people's lives, and seeking a fulfilling and purpose-driven career. It is a profession that not only requires strong medical knowledge and skills but also demands compassion, empathy, and a nurturing spirit. For many, becoming a nurse is not just a job but a deeply meaningful and gratifying life-long vocation.

The different types of nursing programs

- There are several different types of nursing programs, each designed to cater to individuals with varying levels of education and career aspirations. The main types of nursing programs include:

  1. **Certified Nursing Assistant (CNA) Program:**

     - Duration: A few weeks to a few months

     - Description: CNAs provide basic patient care under the supervision of licensed nurses. The program includes fundamental nursing skills, such as assisting with activities of daily living, vital sign measurement, and patient hygiene.

  2. **Licensed Practical Nurse (LPN) Program (or Licensed Vocational Nurse - LVN):**

     - Duration: About 12 to 18 months

     - Description: LPN/LVNs provide more comprehensive patient care under the guidance of registered nurses (RNs) or physicians. They learn practical nursing skills, administer medications, and assist with patient care.

3. **Associate Degree in Nursing (ADN) Program:**

   - Duration: Approximately 2 to 3 years

   - Description: ADN programs are typically offered at community colleges. Graduates are eligible to become registered nurses (RNs) after passing the NCLEX-RN exam. ADN programs focus on nursing fundamentals, basic sciences, and clinical experiences.

4. **Bachelor of Science in Nursing (BSN) Program:**

   - Duration: Around 4 years

   - Description: BSN programs are offered by universities and colleges. Graduates earn a Bachelor's degree in Nursing and are prepared for RN licensure through the NCLEX-RN exam. BSN programs provide a more comprehensive education, including leadership, research, and community health.

5. **Accelerated BSN Programs:**

   - Duration: Typically 12 to 18 months

   - Description: Designed for individuals who already hold a non-nursing Bachelor's degree, accelerated BSN programs offer an intensive and fast-track curriculum to prepare them for RN licensure.

6. **Master of Science in Nursing (MSN) Program:**

   - Duration: About 2 years (after obtaining a BSN)

   - Description: MSN programs are for individuals who wish to specialize in advanced nursing roles, such as nurse practitioner, nurse educator, nurse anesthetist, nurse midwife, or nurse administrator.

7. **Doctor of Nursing Practice (DNP) Program:**

   - Duration: Around 3 to 4 years (after obtaining a BSN or MSN)

   - Description: DNP programs are for advanced practice nurses seeking the highest level of clinical expertise. Graduates often become leaders in healthcare, focusing on evidence-based practice and healthcare improvements.

8. **Ph.D. in Nursing Program:**

   - Duration: Approximately 4 to 5 years (after obtaining a BSN or MSN)

- Description: Ph.D. programs in nursing are research-focused and prepare nurses for careers in academia, research institutions, or leadership positions in healthcare organizations.

Each nursing program has its unique requirements, curriculum, and career outcomes. The choice of program depends on the individual's educational background, career goals, and desired level of nursing practice and responsibility.

The nursing school admissions process

The nursing school admissions process can vary depending on the type of nursing program and the institution offering it. However, there are some common steps and requirements involved in most nursing school admissions processes:

1. **Research and Choose Nursing Programs:** Begin by researching different nursing programs to find the ones that align with your interests, career goals, and educational background. Consider factors such as program type (e.g., ADN, BSN, MSN), location, accreditation, and reputation.

2. **Meet Prerequisite Requirements:** Most nursing programs have specific prerequisite courses that applicants must complete before applying. Common prerequisites include biology, chemistry, anatomy and physiology, nutrition, and psychology. Check with each program for their specific requirements.

3. **Take Standardized Tests:** Some nursing programs require applicants to take standardized tests like the Test of Essential Academic Skills (TEAS) or the Health Education Systems, Inc. (HESI) exam. These tests assess your academic skills in areas relevant to nursing.

4. **Submit Applications:** Complete the application process for the nursing programs you are interested in. This typically involves filling out an online application and paying an application fee.

5. **Write a Personal Statement:** Many nursing programs require applicants to submit a personal statement or essay. Use this opportunity to showcase your passion for nursing, your relevant experiences, and your reasons for pursuing a nursing career.

6. **Obtain Letters of Recommendation:** Some nursing programs may ask for letters of recommendation from teachers, employers, or other individuals who can speak to your character and abilities.

7. **Attend Admissions Interviews (if applicable):** Some nursing programs may require applicants to participate in an admissions interview to assess their communication skills, professionalism, and fit for the program.

8. **Complete Background Checks and Drug Screenings:** Nursing programs

often require applicants to undergo background checks and drug screenings to ensure the safety and well-being of patients.

9. **Wait for Decision Letters:** After submitting your application, you'll need to wait for the nursing programs to review your materials and make a decision. This can take several weeks to a few months, depending on the program.

10. **Acceptance and Enrollment:** If you receive acceptance letters from multiple nursing programs, carefully consider your options and choose the one that best aligns with your goals. Follow the enrollment instructions provided by the school to secure your spot in the program.

11. **Attend Orientation and Begin Nursing School:** Once accepted and enrolled, attend any orientation sessions required by the nursing program. Begin your journey in nursing school, where you will undergo rigorous education and training to become a skilled and compassionate nurse.

It's essential to pay close attention to the deadlines for each nursing program and to follow their specific application instructions. Applying to nursing school can be competitive, so make sure to prepare thoroughly and present yourself in the best possible light throughout the admissions process.

Application costs

The application costs for nursing school can vary depending on the number of schools you apply to, the type of programs you are considering, and other associated expenses. Here are some common costs to consider when applying to nursing school:

1. **Application Fees:** Most nursing schools charge an application fee. The fee amount can vary widely, ranging from around $50 to $150 per application. Some schools may offer fee waivers for students with financial need, so be sure to inquire about this possibility.

2. **Standardized Tests:** If the nursing school requires standardized tests like the Test of Essential Academic Skills (TEAS) or the Health Education Systems, Inc. (HESI) exam, there will be associated costs for registering and taking these tests. The test fees typically range from $50 to $100.

3. **Transcript Fees:** You may need to pay a fee to request and send official transcripts from your previous educational institutions to the nursing schools you are applying to. Transcript fees can vary based on your previous schools' policies.

4. **Additional Application Materials:** Some nursing schools may require additional materials, such as a criminal background check, immunization records, or health screening, which may incur additional costs.

5. **Interview Travel Expenses:** If you are invited for an in-person interview at a

distant nursing school, you may need to cover travel expenses such as transportation, accommodation, and meals.

6. **Preparation Materials:** If you decide to purchase study materials or resources to prepare for admission tests or interviews, there may be associated costs.

7. **Reapplication Costs:** If you decide to reapply to nursing schools in subsequent application cycles, you will need to consider the application fees and any other associated costs again.

It's important to plan ahead and budget for these costs as you prepare to apply to nursing schools. If the application costs are a concern, look into fee waivers, scholarships, or financial assistance programs that may be available to help ease the financial burden. Additionally, consider applying to a mix of nursing schools to increase your chances of acceptance while being mindful of the associated costs.

Chapter 2: Requirements for Nursing School

GPA requirements

- GPA (Grade Point Average) requirements for nursing school admissions can vary widely depending on the type of nursing program and the institution offering it. Different nursing schools may have different minimum GPA requirements, and the competitiveness of the program can also play a role in determining the GPA expectations.

  Here's a general overview of GPA requirements for different types of nursing programs:

  1. **Certified Nursing Assistant (CNA) Program:** CNA programs typically do not have strict GPA requirements. They often focus on providing basic nursing education to individuals without stringent academic prerequisites.

  2. **Licensed Practical Nurse (LPN) Program (or Licensed Vocational Nurse - LVN):** LPN/LVN programs may require a high school diploma or equivalent, but GPA requirements are generally not as demanding as in higher-level nursing programs.

  3. **Associate Degree in Nursing (ADN) Program:** ADN programs typically have GPA requirements ranging from 2.5 to 3.0 on a 4.0 scale. Some more competitive ADN programs may have slightly higher GPA expectations.

  4. **Bachelor of Science in Nursing (BSN) Program:** BSN programs, especially those offered by universities, tend to have higher GPA requirements. GPA expectations for BSN programs can range from 2.75 to 3.5 or higher, depending on the institution.

  5. **Accelerated BSN Programs:** Accelerated BSN programs are designed for individuals who already hold a non-nursing Bachelor's degree. These programs are often competitive, and GPA requirements can be on the higher end, typically ranging from 3.0 to 3.5 or above.

6. **Master of Science in Nursing (MSN) Program:** MSN programs require applicants to have a Bachelor of Science in Nursing (BSN) degree. GPA requirements for MSN programs can vary but generally fall within the range of 3.0 to 3.5 or higher.

It's important to note that while GPA is a significant factor in nursing school admissions, it is not the only criterion considered. Nursing schools also evaluate other aspects of an applicant's profile, such as standardized test scores (if required), prerequisite course completion, letters of recommendation, personal statements, relevant work or volunteer experience, and performance during admissions interviews (if applicable).

If you are interested in applying to nursing school, research the specific GPA requirements for the programs you are considering and work to achieve the best possible GPA during your academic journey. Keep in mind that meeting the minimum GPA requirement does not guarantee admission, especially in competitive programs, so it's essential to present a well-rounded application that showcases your passion for nursing and your commitment to the profession.

Pre-requisites

- Prerequisites, also known as pre-requisites, are specific courses or qualifications that must be completed before a student can be considered for admission into a particular academic program. These requirements ensure that students have the necessary foundational knowledge and skills to succeed in more advanced coursework.

In the context of nursing education, nursing programs often have prerequisite courses that applicants must complete before they can be admitted into the program. These prerequisites vary depending on the type of nursing program (e.g., ADN, BSN, MSN) and the institution offering it. The purpose of nursing prerequisites is to prepare students with a solid academic foundation and the essential knowledge required to thrive in nursing school.

Some common prerequisite courses for nursing programs may include:

1. **Anatomy and Physiology:** A study of the structure and function of the human body.

2. **Microbiology:** The study of microorganisms and their impact on health and disease.

3. **Chemistry:** Basic chemistry principles, often including an emphasis on biochemistry.

4. **Biology:** An introductory course covering various aspects of biology, such as cell biology, genetics, and ecology.

5. **Nutrition:** The study of human nutrition and its role in maintaining health.

6. **Psychology:** An introduction to basic psychology principles and human behavior.

7. **Mathematics:** Depending on the program, some nursing schools may require a college-level math course, often focused on dosage calculations.

8. **English Composition:** A course in academic writing and communication.

It's essential for prospective nursing students to review the specific prerequisites of the nursing programs they are interested in applying to. Some programs may have additional requirements, such as specific grade thresholds for prerequisite courses or certain timeframes within which the courses must have been completed.

Prospective nursing students typically complete their prerequisite courses at a college or university before applying to the nursing program. Once all prerequisites are successfully completed, students can then submit their applications to the nursing school and proceed with the admissions process.

Having a strong academic performance in prerequisite courses can enhance a student's chances of being admitted to their desired nursing program. It is crucial to plan ahead, ensure that all necessary prerequisites are fulfilled, and maintain a competitive academic record to increase the likelihood of successful admission into the nursing program of choice.

The Nursing School Admission Test (NCLEX)

- The National Council Licensure Examination (NCLEX) is a standardized test that is required for licensure as a registered nurse (RN) in the United States and Canada. The NCLEX is a computer-adaptive test (CAT), which means that the difficulty of the questions you are asked is based on your performance on previous questions. This ensures that you are only asked questions that are challenging enough for you to answer correctly.

The NCLEX is divided into two parts: the NCLEX-RN and the NCLEX-PN. The NCLEX-RN is for those who want to become registered nurses, and the NCLEX-PN is for those who want to become licensed practical nurses.

The NCLEX is a challenging test, but it is possible to pass with careful preparation. There are many resources available to help you study for the NCLEX, including practice questions, study guides, and flashcards. You can also find online courses and tutoring services that can help you prepare for the test.

The NCLEX is a vital part of the process of becoming a registered nurse. By passing the NCLEX, you will demonstrate that you have the knowledge and skills necessary to practice safe and effective nursing care.

Here are some additional details about the NCLEX:

- The NCLEX is a 4-hour test, with 75-265 questions.
- The NCLEX is a computer-adaptive test, which means that the difficulty of the questions you are asked is based on your performance on previous questions.
- The passing score for the NCLEX is 75.
- You can take the NCLEX up to 8 times in a 2-year period.
- The NCLEX covers a wide range of nursing topics, including:
    - Health promotion and maintenance
    - Pathophysiology
    - Pharmacology
    - Medical-surgical nursing
    - Maternal-child nursing
    - Pediatric nursing
    - Psychiatric-mental health nursing
    - Nursing research
    - Nursing leadership and management

If you are interested in becoming a registered nurse, the NCLEX is an important step in your journey. By carefully preparing for the test, you can increase your chances of passing and becoming a licensed nurse.

Here are some additional tips for preparing for the NCLEX:

- Start studying early.
- Take practice tests.
- Join a study group.
- Get help from a tutor.
- Stay positive and motivated.

Other requirements

- In addition to GPA requirements and prerequisite courses, nursing schools may have other requirements that applicants must fulfill to be considered for admission. These additional requirements can vary depending on the nursing program and the institution offering it. Some common additional requirements for nursing school admission include:

1. **Health Clearance:** Nursing programs often require applicants to provide evidence of good health and immunization records. This ensures that students can safely participate in clinical experiences and patient care.

2. **Criminal Background Check:** Nursing schools may require applicants to undergo a criminal background check. Certain criminal convictions may impact a student's eligibility for clinical placements and licensure.

3. **Drug Screening:** Nursing schools may require applicants to undergo drug screening to ensure that students are drug-free and can safely care for patients.

4. **CPR Certification:** Many nursing programs require applicants to hold a valid CPR (Cardiopulmonary Resuscitation) certification before starting the program.

5. **Clinical Requirements:** Once accepted into a nursing program, students will participate in clinical experiences at healthcare facilities. Students may need to meet specific clinical requirements, such as health insurance, liability insurance, and compliance with the facility's policies.

6. **Interview:** Some nursing programs conduct interviews as part of the admissions process. The interview allows the school to assess an applicant's communication skills, professionalism, and motivation for pursuing a career in nursing.

7. **Relevant Experience:** While not always mandatory, relevant healthcare experience, such as volunteering or working as a nursing assistant, can strengthen an applicant's profile and demonstrate their commitment to the field.

8. **English Language Proficiency:** For applicants whose first language is not English, some nursing programs may require proof of English language proficiency, such as TOEFL or IELTS scores.

9. **Essays or Personal Statements:** Nursing schools may request essays or personal statements from applicants to gain insight into their motivations, aspirations, and commitment to nursing.

It's crucial for prospective nursing students to carefully review the specific admission requirements of the nursing programs they are interested in applying to. Meeting all the requirements and submitting a complete and well-prepared application can increase an applicant's chances of being accepted into their desired nursing program. Additionally, staying organized and attentive to deadlines is essential throughout the application process.

Chapter 3: Preparing Your Application

Choosing the right schools

Choosing the right nursing schools is a crucial decision that can significantly impact your nursing education and future career. Here are some essential factors to consider when selecting nursing schools:

1. **Accreditation:** Ensure that the nursing programs you are considering are accredited by recognized accrediting bodies. Accreditation ensures that the school meets certain standards of quality education and will be essential for obtaining licensure and future career opportunities.

2. **Program Type and Level:** Determine the type of nursing program you want to pursue (e.g., ADN, BSN, MSN) and the level of education you wish to achieve. Different nursing programs offer varying levels of education and specialization options.

3. **Location:** Consider the location of the nursing school. Are you willing to relocate for your nursing education, or do you prefer schools within your local area? Consider factors such as proximity to family, cost of living, and potential clinical placement opportunities.

4. **Cost and Financial Aid:** Evaluate the tuition and other associated costs of attending the nursing program. Look into the availability of financial aid, scholarships, or grants to help offset the expenses.

5. **NCLEX Pass Rates:** Research the NCLEX pass rates of the nursing programs you are interested in. High NCLEX pass rates indicate that the program prepares students well for the licensing exam.

6. **Clinical Opportunities:** Find out the types of clinical experiences offered by the nursing school and the range of healthcare facilities where students may have clinical rotations. Diverse clinical experiences can enhance your learning and exposure to different nursing specialties.

7. **Faculty and Resources:** Investigate the qualifications and experience of the nursing faculty. Faculty expertise and student-to-faculty ratios can impact the

quality of education you receive. Additionally, consider the availability of resources such as simulation labs, libraries, and tutoring services.

8. **Specializations and Electives:** If you have a particular nursing specialization in mind, check if the nursing school offers relevant specialty tracks or electives. Some schools may have strengths in specific nursing areas.

9. **Campus Culture and Support Services:** Visit the campuses if possible or research online to get a sense of the school's culture and support services. Look for schools that prioritize student success and well-being.

10. **Career Services:** Investigate the nursing school's career services and job placement support. A strong career services department can assist you in finding internships, residencies, and job opportunities after graduation.

11. **Alumni Network:** Check if the nursing school has an active alumni network. Networking with alumni can provide valuable insights, mentorship, and potential job connections.

12. **Ratings and Reviews:** Read reviews and ratings of the nursing schools from current students and alumni to gain additional perspectives on the program's strengths and weaknesses.

Remember to prioritize your individual goals, preferences, and needs when choosing nursing schools. Make a list of the schools that align with your criteria, and if possible, visit the campuses or attend virtual open houses to get a firsthand feel of the environment. By carefully considering these factors, you can make an informed decision and choose a nursing school that will help you achieve your career aspirations in the nursing profession.

Completing the application

Completing the application for nursing school is a crucial step in the admissions process. Here's a general overview of the steps involved in completing the application:

1. **Review Application Requirements:** Carefully read through the nursing school's application requirements and instructions. Make a checklist of all the documents, forms, and information you need to submit.

2. **Create an Account (if applicable):** Some nursing schools may require you to create an online account to start the application process. Follow the provided instructions to set up your account.

3. **Personal Information:** Provide your personal details, including your full name, contact information, date of birth, and address.

4. **Educational Background:** List all your previous educational institutions, including high school and any colleges or universities you attended. Enter the names, dates attended, and degrees earned.

5. **Transcripts:** Request official transcripts from all previous educational institutions you attended. Nursing schools typically require transcripts as proof of completion of prerequisite courses and academic performance.

6. **Prerequisite Coursework:** Indicate the prerequisite courses you have completed or are currently taking. Some applications may ask for specific grades or GPA in these courses.

7. **Standardized Test Scores (if applicable):** If the nursing school requires standardized test scores, such as the TEAS or HESI exam, provide the relevant scores or arrange to have them sent to the school.

8. **Essays or Personal Statements:** If the application requires an essay or personal statement, compose a well-written piece that showcases your passion for nursing, relevant experiences, and reasons for applying to the program.

9. **Letters of Recommendation:** If the nursing school requires letters of recommendation, request them from teachers, employers, or other individuals who can speak to your academic abilities and character.

10. **Application Fee:** Pay the required application fee, if applicable. Some nursing schools charge an application fee to process your application.

11. **Submit the Application:** Review your completed application to ensure all the information is accurate and complete. Submit the application through the school's designated application portal or mail it to the specified address.

12. **Follow Up:** After submitting your application, follow up with the nursing school to ensure they have received all required documents and that your application is complete.

13. **Admissions Interview (if applicable):** Some nursing schools may invite selected applicants for an admissions interview. If you are asked to participate in an interview, prepare for it thoroughly and be ready to discuss your interest in nursing and your academic goals.

14. **Wait for Decision:** Once you have submitted your application and completed any required interviews, wait for the nursing school to review your application. Admission decisions are typically communicated by mail or email within a specified timeframe.

Remember to meet all application deadlines and provide accurate and truthful information throughout the application process. Completing the application thoroughly and on time will increase your chances of being considered for admission to the nursing school of your choice.

Writing your personal statement

Writing a compelling personal statement is a crucial part of the nursing school application process. This is your opportunity to showcase your passion for nursing, your experiences, and your unique qualities that make you a strong candidate for the program. Here are some tips to help you write an effective personal statement:

1. **Be Genuine and Personal:** Share your genuine reasons for wanting to become a nurse. Explain what motivates you to pursue a career in nursing and how your personal experiences have influenced your decision.

2. **Tell a Story:** Instead of listing achievements or qualities, weave your experiences and aspirations into a compelling narrative. Use anecdotes or real-life examples to make your statement engaging and memorable.

3. **Highlight Relevant Experiences:** Discuss any relevant experiences you've had in healthcare, volunteering, or caregiving. Explain how these experiences have shaped your understanding of nursing and influenced your desire to become a nurse.

4. **Showcase Your Strengths:** Highlight your strengths and attributes that align with the qualities of a successful nurse. This could include empathy, problem-solving skills, adaptability, and effective communication.

5. **Connect to the Program:** Research the nursing program and find specific aspects that resonate with you. Mention why you believe this program is the right fit for your nursing education and career goals.

6. **Address Weaknesses (if applicable):** If there are any weaknesses in your application, such as lower grades in certain courses, briefly address them in your statement. Explain any extenuating circumstances and focus on how you've learned and grown from those experiences.

7. **Be Concise and Clear:** Keep your personal statement focused and concise. Adhere to any word or page limits specified by the nursing school.

8. **Proofread and Edit:** Carefully proofread your personal statement to eliminate any grammatical errors or typos. Ask friends, family, or teachers to review it for feedback and suggestions.

9. **Use Professional Language:** Write in a professional and formal tone. Avoid slang, jargon, or overly casual language.

10. **Be Positive and Enthusiastic:** Convey your enthusiasm for nursing and your commitment to making a difference in patients' lives. Positive energy can make a lasting impression on the admissions committee.

11. **Start Early:** Give yourself plenty of time to brainstorm, write, and revise your personal statement. Starting early will allow you to craft a well-thought-out and

polished statement.

12. **Avoid Clichés:** Avoid using clichés or overly generic statements. Instead, focus on original thoughts and personal insights.

Remember, your personal statement is an opportunity to showcase your personality, aspirations, and dedication to the nursing profession. Be sincere, thoughtful, and passionate in your writing. A strong personal statement can make a significant difference in your nursing school application, so take the time to make it shine!

Example

As a young child, I was fascinated by the human body and drawn to the idea of helping others. Growing up in a family where healthcare was valued and respected, I witnessed the compassionate care my grandmother received from nurses during her battle with cancer. Those experiences instilled in me a profound appreciation for the nursing profession and inspired my unwavering desire to become a nurse.

I believe that nursing is not merely a career but a calling to serve and advocate for those in need. Throughout my academic journey, I have been diligently working towards this dream. My dedication to academic excellence has led me to achieve top grades in science and math courses, laying the foundation for my pursuit of a nursing degree. However, it is my experiences beyond the classroom that have solidified my commitment to nursing.

For the past two years, I have volunteered at a local hospice, providing companionship and emotional support to terminally ill patients and their families. Witnessing the profound impact a caring presence can have on someone facing the end of life has reinforced my belief in the power of empathy and human connection. These experiences have taught me that being a nurse is not just about administering medications and treatments but about being a source of comfort and strength for patients and their loved ones during their most vulnerable moments.

I am particularly drawn to your esteemed nursing program because of its reputation for excellence in patient-centered care and community outreach. The emphasis on hands-on clinical experiences and opportunities to work with diverse patient populations aligns perfectly with my goal to become a well-rounded and compassionate nurse.

Throughout my journey to nursing, I have also developed strong communication skills, adaptability, and the ability to work effectively in a team. These qualities were further honed during my time as a volunteer EMT, where I learned to think critically under pressure and respond to medical emergencies with composure and efficiency.

As a future nurse, I am committed to lifelong learning and staying abreast of the latest advancements in healthcare. I envision myself actively engaging in evidence-based practice and contributing to the improvement of patient outcomes and the nursing profession as a whole.

In conclusion, my passion for nursing is not merely a fleeting aspiration; it is the guiding force that has directed my path and continues to drive my commitment to the art and science of nursing. I am excited to embark on this transformative journey with your esteemed nursing program and humbly request the opportunity to contribute my dedication, empathy, and unwavering commitment to the nursing profession.

Please remember that this is just an example, and your personal statement should reflect your unique experiences, motivations, and aspirations. Tailor your statement to genuinely express your passion for nursing and what makes you a strong candidate for the nursing school you are applying to. Good luck with your application!

Getting letters of recommendation

Getting strong letters of recommendation is an essential part of your nursing school application. These letters provide valuable insights into your character, abilities, and potential as a future nurse. Here's a step-by-step guide to obtaining effective letters of recommendation:

1. **Choose the Right Recommenders:** Select individuals who can speak to your academic performance, work ethic, clinical skills, and personal qualities. Ideal recommenders include professors, supervisors, healthcare professionals, or volunteer coordinators who know you well and can provide meaningful insights into your qualifications for nursing school.

2. **Ask Early and Politely:** Approach potential recommenders well in advance of the application deadline. Send a polite email or schedule a meeting to discuss your request. Be considerate of their time and workload.

3. **Provide Relevant Information:** Give your recommenders all the necessary information to write a compelling letter. Provide them with your updated resume, a summary of your academic and extracurricular achievements, and a copy of your personal statement. This will help them tailor the letter to your nursing aspirations.

4. **Remind Them of Your Accomplishments:** Briefly remind your recommenders of any specific projects or experiences you had together that highlight your strengths and suitability for nursing school.

5. **Discuss Your Goals:** Share your career goals and why nursing is essential to you. This will help your recommenders understand your motivations and tailor their letters accordingly.

6. **Follow Up Politely:** If your recommenders agree to write the letters, follow up with a thank-you note expressing your appreciation for their support. Provide

gentle reminders as the deadline approaches, but avoid being pushy.

7. **Waive Your Right to Read:** Many recommenders prefer to write confidential letters, so consider waiving your right to read the letters. This shows trust in their judgment and ensures that the recommendations are sincere.

8. **Provide Clear Submission Instructions:** Inform your recommenders of the submission process and any specific requirements of the nursing school. This includes details such as whether the letters should be submitted online, through email, or mailed directly to the school.

9. **Stay Organized:** Keep track of the submission deadlines for each nursing school and ensure that your recommenders have enough time to meet them. Create a checklist to monitor your progress.

10. **Express Gratitude:** After you are admitted to a nursing program, be sure to thank your recommenders for their support. Consider sending a thoughtful note or small token of appreciation.

Remember that the letters of recommendation provide a third-party perspective on your abilities, character, and potential as a nurse. Choose recommenders who can speak positively about your qualifications and dedication to the nursing profession. Personalized and sincere recommendations can strengthen your nursing school application and increase your chances of being accepted into the program of your choice.

What about Internships, or observational experiences

Internships, observational experiences, or working as an aide to observe and assist nurses can be incredibly valuable in preparing for nursing school and enhancing your nursing school application. These experiences provide you with firsthand exposure to the nursing profession, allowing you to gain insights into the daily responsibilities of nurses and the healthcare environment. They can also help you develop essential skills and qualities that will benefit you during nursing school and in your future nursing career. Here's how these experiences can be beneficial:

1. **Insight into the Nursing Profession:** Internships or observational experiences allow you to witness nursing in action and understand the various roles nurses play in patient care. You'll gain a deeper appreciation for the profession and confirm your interest in pursuing nursing as a career.

2. **Clinical Skills Development:** By assisting nurses and observing their work, you can learn and practice basic clinical skills, such as taking vital signs, providing basic patient care, and assisting with activities of daily living. These skills can give you a head start when you enter nursing school.

3. **Communication and Interpersonal Skills:** Working with patients, healthcare

professionals, and other staff members helps you hone your communication and interpersonal skills. Effective communication is crucial in nursing, and these experiences allow you to develop rapport and empathy with patients and their families.

4. **Exposure to Diverse Healthcare Settings:** Internships or observational experiences may take place in various healthcare settings, such as hospitals, clinics, long-term care facilities, or community health centers. This exposure helps you understand the different aspects of healthcare and the diverse patient populations nurses serve.

5. **Networking Opportunities:** Building relationships with nurses and healthcare professionals during these experiences can provide valuable networking opportunities. These connections may prove helpful in the future for advice, mentorship, or even job opportunities.

6. **Enhanced Nursing School Application:** Including your experiences as an intern or healthcare aide in your nursing school application can strengthen your application. Admissions committees appreciate applicants who have actively sought out experiences in the field to demonstrate their commitment to nursing.

7. **Increased Confidence:** Engaging in practical experiences before nursing school can boost your confidence in your decision to pursue nursing. It can also make you feel more prepared to handle the challenges of nursing school and clinical rotations.

Keep in mind that while these experiences can be beneficial, they are not typically mandatory for nursing school admission. However, they can significantly enhance your understanding of nursing and your readiness for the nursing school curriculum. If you have the opportunity to participate in internships, shadowing experiences, or work as a healthcare aide, seize the chance to learn and grow as a future nurse. Remember to reflect on these experiences in your personal statement or interviews to showcase the impact they had on your decision to pursue nursing as a career.

Chapter 4: Interviewing for Nursing School

What to expect

Interviewing for nursing school is a critical step in the admissions process. It allows the nursing program's admissions committee to get to know you better beyond what's on your application. Here's what you can expect during a nursing school interview:

1. **Format:** Nursing school interviews can take various formats. Some may be one-on-one interviews with a faculty member or an admissions committee member, while others may be group interviews with multiple applicants.

2. **Location:** Interviews may be conducted in person on the school's campus, via video conference, or over the phone, depending on the circumstances and the school's preferences.

3. **Duration:** Interviews generally last anywhere from 15 minutes to 30 minutes, although the exact duration can vary.

4. **Types of Questions:** The questions asked during the interview are designed to assess your suitability for nursing school and your passion for the profession. Expect a mix of behavioral questions (e.g., "Tell us about a challenging situation you faced and how you handled it?") and questions that probe your understanding of nursing (e.g., "What do you think are the most critical qualities of a nurse?").

5. **Academic Background:** Be prepared to discuss your academic background, including any relevant coursework, extracurricular activities, and your GPA. They may ask about specific courses or experiences mentioned in your application.

6. **Motivation for Nursing:** You'll likely be asked about why you chose nursing as a career and what motivates you to become a nurse. Be sincere and share your passion for helping others and your desire to make a positive impact on patients' lives.

7. **Strengths and Weaknesses:** Be ready to talk about your strengths and how they align with the qualities of a successful nurse. You may also be asked about areas where you feel you need improvement.

8. **Knowledge of the Nursing Profession:** Prepare by researching the nursing profession and current healthcare issues. Demonstrating your understanding of the nursing field shows your commitment and dedication to the profession.

9. **Questions for the Interviewers:** At the end of the interview, you'll likely have the opportunity to ask questions. Prepare thoughtful questions about the nursing program, clinical opportunities, or any other aspects you want to know more about.

10. **Professionalism and Communication:** During the interview, dress professionally, maintain good eye contact, and speak clearly and confidently. Demonstrate your ability to communicate effectively, as this is a crucial skill in nursing.

Remember that the interview is a chance for the nursing school to get to know you as a person and assess whether you'll be a good fit for their program. Be authentic, showcase your genuine passion for nursing, and demonstrate your dedication to becoming a compassionate and competent nurse. Practice with mock interviews or with a friend or family member to help you feel more confident and prepared. Good luck with your nursing school interview!

How to prepare

Preparing for a nursing school interview requires careful research, self-reflection, and practice. Here are some tips to help you get ready for your interview:

1. **Research the Nursing Program:** Familiarize yourself with the nursing school you are interviewing with. Know their mission, values, and unique aspects of their program. Understand the curriculum, clinical opportunities, and any specializations they offer.

2. **Review Your Application Materials:** Revisit your application, personal statement, and resume to remind yourself of the experiences, achievements, and qualities you highlighted. Be prepared to discuss them in more detail during the interview.

3. **Know Nursing Basics:** Refresh your knowledge of essential nursing concepts, healthcare trends, and challenges in the nursing profession. Stay informed about current healthcare issues and how they relate to nursing practice.

4. **Practice Common Interview Questions:** Prepare responses to common nursing school interview questions, such as your reasons for choosing nursing, strengths and weaknesses, examples of teamwork or leadership experiences, and how you handle challenges.

5. **Reflect on Your Experiences:** Think about your healthcare-related experiences, whether through volunteer work, shadowing, or previous jobs.

Reflect on how these experiences shaped your desire to become a nurse and what you learned from them.

6. **Research Ethical Scenarios:** Be ready to discuss ethical dilemmas that nurses may face. Think critically about how you would respond to situations that involve patient confidentiality, moral dilemmas, or challenging patient interactions.

7. **Know Your Long-Term Goals:** Consider your long-term career goals in nursing and how the nursing school's program aligns with them. Show that you have thought about your future as a nurse.

8. **Practice Communication Skills:** Strong communication is essential for nurses. Practice articulating your thoughts clearly and confidently. Pay attention to your body language and maintain good eye contact during the interview.

9. **Mock Interviews:** Conduct mock interviews with friends, family, or career advisors. Practice answering questions and receiving feedback on your responses.

10. **Prepare Questions to Ask:** Think of thoughtful questions to ask the interviewers at the end of the interview. Inquiring about the nursing program's strengths, clinical experiences, or alumni outcomes demonstrates your interest in the school.

11. **Review Interview Logistics:** Know the interview format, location (if in-person), and any technical requirements (if online). Test any video conferencing tools in advance to avoid last-minute technical issues.

12. **Plan Your Attire:** Dress professionally and appropriately for the interview. Choose attire that aligns with the nursing profession's standards of professionalism.

13. **Be Yourself:** Be authentic and genuine during the interview. Let your passion for nursing and your commitment to patient care shine through your responses.

Remember that an interview is an opportunity for the nursing school to learn more about you beyond your application. Be confident, showcase your strengths, and express your enthusiasm for nursing. By thoroughly preparing and being yourself, you can increase your chances of making a positive impression and securing a spot in the nursing program. Good luck with your interview!

What to wear

When choosing what to wear for a nursing school interview, it's essential to dress professionally and appropriately to make a positive impression. Here are some guidelines on what to wear:

1. **Business Professional Attire:** Opt for business professional attire, as it conveys a sense of professionalism and respect for the interview process. This

dress code typically includes:

- Men: A well-fitted suit in a neutral color such as navy, gray, or black. Pair it with a dress shirt, a conservative tie, dark-colored dress shoes, and dark socks.
- Women: A tailored suit with a blazer and matching pants or a knee-length skirt. Wear a conservative blouse or button-down shirt underneath. Choose closed-toe, low-heeled dress shoes.

2. **Avoid Casual Attire:** Avoid wearing casual clothing, such as jeans, t-shirts, sneakers, or flip-flops. Dressing too casually may give the impression of not taking the interview seriously.

3. **Neat and Clean Appearance:** Ensure your clothing is clean, wrinkle-free, and well-groomed. Pay attention to personal hygiene and avoid strong perfumes or colognes.

4. **Minimal Accessories:** Keep accessories simple and professional. Avoid flashy jewelry or accessories that may be distracting.

5. **Comfortable Dress Shoes:** Wear comfortable and polished dress shoes that you can walk comfortably in. Avoid high heels that might cause discomfort during the interview.

6. **Nails and Hair:** Ensure your nails are clean and well-groomed. If you have long hair, consider tying it back neatly to keep it from falling into your face during the interview.

7. **Tattoos and Piercings:** If you have visible tattoos or multiple piercings, consider covering or removing them for the interview, if possible. Some nursing schools may have specific dress code policies.

8. **Observe the School Culture:** If you know the nursing school's culture and dress code, try to align your attire accordingly. Some schools may have specific guidelines or preferences.

Remember, dressing professionally shows that you take the nursing school interview seriously and that you are prepared to represent yourself as a future healthcare professional. It's always better to be slightly overdressed than underdressed for such occasions. Taking the time to dress appropriately will help you make a positive first impression during your nursing school interview.

What to say

During a nursing school interview, what you say plays a significant role in showcasing your qualifications, passion for nursing, and suitability for the program. Here are some key points to cover and tips on what to say during the interview:

1. **Express Your Passion for Nursing:** Start by conveying your genuine enthusiasm for nursing and your desire to make a positive impact on patients' lives. Explain what drew you to the nursing profession and why you are committed to pursuing a career in healthcare.

2. **Discuss Relevant Experiences:** Highlight any healthcare-related experiences you've had, such as volunteering, shadowing, or working as a healthcare aide. Describe what you learned from these experiences and how they reinforced your interest in nursing.

3. **Showcase Your Strengths:** Talk about your strengths and how they align with the qualities of an effective nurse. Emphasize traits like compassion, empathy, strong communication skills, problem-solving abilities, and a commitment to lifelong learning.

4. **Address Your Academic Background:** Be prepared to discuss your academic achievements, coursework, and any challenges you may have overcome. If there are any areas of your academic history that need clarification, explain them briefly and focus on how you have improved and learned from those experiences.

5. **Demonstrate Your Understanding of the Nursing Profession:** Show that you have researched the nursing profession and understand its responsibilities, challenges, and the importance of teamwork in healthcare settings.

6. **Share Your Long-Term Goals:** Discuss your aspirations beyond nursing school, such as pursuing advanced degrees, specializing in a particular area of nursing, or engaging in research or advocacy.

7. **Reflect on Ethical Scenarios:** Be ready to discuss ethical dilemmas that nurses may encounter and how you would approach them. Demonstrate your ability to think critically and ethically about patient care.

8. **Ask Thoughtful Questions:** At the end of the interview, ask insightful questions about the nursing program, clinical experiences, faculty support, or any other aspects you are curious about. This shows your interest and engagement in the program.

9. **Maintain Professionalism:** Speak clearly and confidently. Avoid using slang or informal language. Be polite and respectful to the interviewers.

10. **Be Genuine and Authentic:** Be yourself during the interview. Authenticity is crucial, and interviewers appreciate sincerity and honesty.

11. **Practice Active Listening:** Pay close attention to the questions asked by the interviewers and respond thoughtfully. Take a moment to gather your thoughts before answering if needed.

12. **Thank the Interviewers:** At the end of the interview, express your gratitude for the opportunity to interview and thank the interviewers for their time and consideration.

Remember that the interview is a chance for you to demonstrate your potential as a nursing student and future healthcare professional. Stay positive, confident, and composed throughout the interview. Practicing mock interviews beforehand can help you feel more comfortable and prepared for the actual interview. Good luck with your nursing school interview!

Chapter 5: Getting Accepted to Nursing School

The waiting game

The waiting period after submitting your nursing school application can be both exciting and nerve-wracking. Here are some tips on how to handle the waiting game:

1. **Stay Positive:** It's natural to feel anxious during the waiting period, but try to stay positive and confident in your abilities. Remind yourself of the hard work you put into your application and trust that you presented yourself well.

2. **Engage in Meaningful Activities:** Keep yourself busy with meaningful activities during the waiting period. Focus on your studies, volunteer work, or other hobbies that you enjoy. Engaging in activities you are passionate about can help distract you from the waiting and reduce stress.

3. **Avoid Overthinking:** Try not to overanalyze or obsessively think about the outcome of your application. Instead, focus on what you can control in the present.

4. **Reach Out for Updates (if Appropriate):** If the nursing school provides updates on the application status, follow their guidelines for reaching out. However, avoid excessive inquiries that may be seen as impatience.

5. **Prepare for Next Steps:** Take this time to prepare for potential next steps, such as the interview, if applicable. Review common interview questions and practice your responses.

6. **Connect with Others:** Reach out to friends or family who may have gone through a similar experience or are supportive of your nursing aspirations. Talking to others can help alleviate some of the stress.

7. **Take Care of Yourself:** Practice self-care during the waiting period. Get enough rest, eat well, exercise, and engage in activities that help you relax and recharge.

8. **Visualize Success:** Imagine yourself succeeding and getting accepted into the nursing program. Positive visualization can boost your confidence and reduce anxiety.

9. **Remember It's Not Personal:** Keep in mind that the admissions process is

competitive, and the decision is not a reflection of your worth as an individual. Admission decisions are often based on a variety of factors, and the outcome is not entirely within your control.

10. **Plan for Alternatives:** While you hope for the best, it's essential to be prepared for different outcomes. Consider alternative options or other nursing programs you may be interested in if your first-choice school doesn't work out.

11. **Celebrate Your Achievements:** Acknowledge your efforts and accomplishments throughout the application process. Regardless of the outcome, going through the application process is an achievement in itself.

Remember that waiting for the nursing school decision is a temporary phase, and soon you will have clarity on the outcome. Stay patient, stay positive, and trust in your abilities. Your dedication and passion for nursing will undoubtedly lead you to the right path, no matter the result.

What to do if you're not accepted

If you're not accepted into a nursing school, it can be disheartening, but it's essential to stay positive and proactive. Here are some steps to take if you find yourself in this situation:

1. **Stay Positive and Don't Get Discouraged:** Remember that not being accepted does not define your worth or potential as a nurse. Stay positive and maintain confidence in your abilities and passion for nursing.

2. **Seek Feedback (if Available):** If the nursing school offers feedback on your application, take advantage of the opportunity to learn more about areas for improvement. Understanding the reasons for the decision can help you strengthen your future applications.

3. **Consider Alternative Nursing Programs:** Research other nursing schools or programs that may align with your interests and career goals. Different schools have different admission criteria, and you may find a better fit elsewhere.

4. **Explore Different Paths:** Consider other healthcare-related career options or related fields that interest you. There are various roles in the healthcare industry where your skills and passion for helping others can be utilized.

5. **Gain More Experience:** Use the time to gain additional healthcare-related experience through volunteering, shadowing, or working as a healthcare aide. Building a diverse and robust portfolio can enhance your future applications.

6. **Upgrade Your Skills and Knowledge:** Take advantage of the time to improve your academic performance or retake prerequisite courses to enhance your academic qualifications.

7. **Meet with an Advisor or Counselor:** Speak with an academic advisor or

counselor to discuss your options and create a plan for reapplication or exploring alternative paths.

8. **Consider Transfer Options:** If you are attending a community college, consider the possibility of transferring to a four-year nursing program after completing prerequisites and gaining relevant experience.

9. **Stay Committed to Your Goals:** Reflect on your passion for nursing and reaffirm your commitment to pursuing this career. Keep your long-term goals in mind as you navigate your next steps.

10. **Network and Seek Support:** Connect with others in the nursing field, join online nursing communities, or attend nursing-related events to build connections and gather advice and support.

11. **Reapply in the Future:** If nursing remains your passion, don't be discouraged from reapplying to nursing schools in the future. Use the time to strengthen your application and demonstrate growth.

12. **Consider Other Opportunities:** Explore alternative paths within the healthcare field or related fields that interest you. There are various rewarding careers in healthcare beyond nursing.

Remember that setbacks are a natural part of life, and they can present opportunities for growth and learning. Use this experience as motivation to become an even stronger candidate for nursing school or explore other fulfilling paths in healthcare. With determination, perseverance, and a positive attitude, you can work towards achieving your goals and aspirations.

Next steps

The next steps after not being accepted into a nursing school will depend on your individual goals, circumstances, and preferences. Here are some general next steps you can consider:

1. **Evaluate Your Options:** Take some time to carefully evaluate your options. Reflect on your passion for nursing and whether you want to pursue other healthcare-related careers or explore different fields of study.

2. **Reevaluate Your Nursing School Choices:** If you are committed to becoming a nurse, reconsider your nursing school choices. Look into other nursing programs that may be a better fit for your qualifications and aspirations.

3. **Strengthen Your Application:** Use the time to enhance your application for future nursing school admissions. Focus on improving your academic performance, gaining more healthcare experience, and obtaining strong letters of recommendation.

4. **Continue Gaining Healthcare Experience:** Continue volunteering, shadowing,

or working in healthcare settings to expand your knowledge and skills and demonstrate your commitment to the field.

5. **Seek Academic Support:** If you struggled with certain prerequisite courses, consider seeking academic support, such as tutoring or academic advising, to help you excel in those areas.

6. **Consider Transferring:** If you are attending a community college or another institution, explore transfer options to nursing programs at other colleges or universities.

7. **Explore Related Healthcare Careers:** Research other healthcare professions that align with your interests and strengths. Consider fields such as medical assisting, occupational therapy, medical laboratory technology, or public health.

8. **Speak with Advisors or Counselors:** Seek guidance from academic advisors, career counselors, or mentors. They can provide valuable insights and help you navigate your options.

9. **Continue Learning and Growing:** Engage in continuous learning and personal development. Pursue relevant courses, certifications, or workshops to enhance your skills and knowledge.

10. **Stay Positive and Persistent:** The path to achieving your goals may have some twists and turns. Stay positive, persistent, and open to exploring new opportunities.

11. **Network and Connect:** Build connections within the healthcare community. Networking can lead to new opportunities and valuable advice from professionals in the field.

12. **Celebrate Your Progress:** Acknowledge the effort and progress you make along your journey. Every step you take brings you closer to your goals.

Remember that setbacks are a natural part of life, and sometimes they can lead to unexpected opportunities and growth. Stay committed to your aspirations, remain proactive in pursuing your passions, and be open to exploring different paths. Your determination and dedication will guide you towards a fulfilling and rewarding career, whether it's in nursing or another field that aligns with your interests and strengths.

Anything else I should know about how to apply and get admitted to nursing school?

Absolutely! Here are some additional tips and important things to consider when applying and striving to get admitted to nursing school:

1. **Research Multiple Nursing Schools:** Explore various nursing schools and programs to find the ones that align with your interests, career goals, and preferences. Consider factors such as program reputation, accreditation, faculty expertise, clinical opportunities, and location.

2. **Admission Requirements and Deadlines:** Review each nursing school's admission requirements, prerequisites, and application deadlines carefully. Start preparing well in advance to ensure you meet all the requirements on time.

3. **Consider Different Program Levels:** Nursing programs offer different levels of education, such as Associate Degree in Nursing (ADN), Bachelor of Science in Nursing (BSN), and Master of Science in Nursing (MSN). Choose the program that best suits your career goals and timeline.

4. **Maintain a Competitive GPA:** Academic performance is crucial for nursing school admission. Work hard to maintain a competitive GPA, especially in science and prerequisite courses.

5. **Volunteer and Gain Experience:** Participate in healthcare-related volunteer work, internships, or healthcare aide positions to gain relevant experience and demonstrate your commitment to the nursing profession.

6. **Prepare for Nursing Admission Tests:** Some nursing schools require admission tests like the TEAS or HESI. Study and prepare well for these tests to achieve competitive scores.

7. **Letters of Recommendation:** Seek strong letters of recommendation from individuals who can attest to your academic abilities, work ethic, and suitability for nursing.

8. **Personal Statement:** Craft a compelling personal statement that showcases your passion for nursing, relevant experiences, and qualities that make you a strong candidate.

9. **Meet Prerequisite Requirements:** Ensure you complete all prerequisite courses required for the nursing program you're applying to. Check if any courses have expiration dates.

10. **Stay Organized:** Keep track of application deadlines, requirements, and submission status for each nursing school. Be proactive and submit all materials well before the deadline.

11. **Be Adaptable and Open-Minded:** Be prepared for the possibility of not getting into your top-choice nursing school. Consider alternative options and be open to exploring different nursing programs.

12. **Interview Preparation:** If the nursing school requires an interview, practice mock interviews with friends or family to build your confidence and refine your responses.

13. **Financial Planning:** Consider the cost of nursing school and explore financial aid options, scholarships, and grants to help fund your education.

14. **Attend Information Sessions:** Participate in nursing school information sessions, open houses, or virtual events to learn more about the program and connect with faculty and current students.

15. **Demonstrate Commitment to Nursing:** Show your dedication to the nursing profession through consistent involvement in healthcare-related activities and a genuine passion for patient care.

Applying to nursing school can be a competitive process, but with careful preparation, dedication, and a genuine passion for nursing, you can increase your chances of getting admitted to the nursing program of your dreams. Remember to be persistent and resilient throughout the process. Best of luck on your journey to becoming a nurse!

This is just a general outline, and the specific requirements and process will vary depending on the nursing school. However, this should give you a good overview of what you need to do to apply and get admitted to nursing school.

Here are some additional tips that may help you on your journey to becoming a nurse:

- Start early. The process of getting into nursing school can take several years, so it is important to start early. This will give you time to complete the necessary coursework, take the NCLEX, and gain relevant experience.

- Get good grades. Your GPA is one of the most important factors in nursing school admissions. Aim for a GPA of 3.7 or higher.

- Take the NCLEX. The NCLEX is a standardized test that is required for admission to nursing school. It is important to score well on the NCLEX, as your score will be compared to other applicants.

- Gain relevant experience. Nursing schools want to see that you are committed to a career in nursing. Gain relevant experience by shadowing nurses, volunteering in a medical setting, or conducting research.

- Write a strong personal statement. Your personal statement is your chance to tell the admissions committee why you want to be a nurse. Make sure your statement is well-written and that it highlights your strengths and experiences.

- Get strong letters of recommendation. Letters of recommendation are an important part of your nursing school application. Ask professors, mentors, or other professionals who know you well to write letters on your behalf.

- Apply to a variety of schools. Nursing school admissions is a competitive process, so it is important to apply to a variety of schools. This will increase your chances of getting accepted.